SARRA CHENIK
AYMEN NOAMEN

Practical aspects of setting up a cardio-oncology unit

SARRA CHENIK
AYMEN NOAMEN

Practical aspects of setting up a cardio-oncology unit

project for the cardiology department of the Tunis military hospital

ScienciaScripts

Imprint

Cover image: www.ingimage.com

This book is a translation from the original published under ISBN 978-620-3-44283-0.

Publisher:
Sciencia Scripts
is a trademark of
Dodo Books Indian Ocean Ltd. and OmniScriptum S.R.L publishing group

120 High Road, East Finchley, London, N2 9ED, United Kingdom
Str. Armeneasca 28/1, office 1, Chisinau MD-2012, Republic of Moldova, Europe
Printed at: see last page
ISBN: 978-620-6-22276-7

Contents

Introduction

Worldwide, the five-year survival of cancer patients is estimated at 43.2 million [1]. The development of new cancer treatments has improved the survival of cancer patients, which is why cancer has often become a chronic disease. Unfortunately, these anti-cancer treatments are not without undesirable effects, particularly cardiovascular. Cardiovascular side-effects are very common in this group of patients. Chemotherapy, hormonal therapy, radiotherapy and new, more targeted therapies such as immunotherapy are all associated with multiple cardiac and vascular complications that are often poorly understood [2]. What's more, these complications sometimes occur months or even years after treatment, which is an additional difficulty. Cardio-oncology (or onco-cardiology) arose in the 1970s from observations of patients who developed heart failure after being treated with anthracyclines. The term was coined in 1996. Its development has accelerated since the early 2000s with the creation of dedicated clinical units, the first by D. Cardinale in Milan in 2009 and, in France, in Marseille in 2013. At the Georges Pompidou European Hospital in Paris, one of the themes of the university hospital department set up in 2012 was cardio-oncology. At the same time, the creation in 2009 of an international learned society, a specialist journal, dedicated sessions at cardiology and oncology congresses and an explosion in publications reflect the reality and growing importance of the problem. Cardiovascular disease is more frequent and more serious in cancer patients than in the general population, and these patients, who are becoming increasingly numerous, are not being managed optimally, due to a lack of appropriate organisation and dedicated research.

Cardiovascular mortality in cancer patients is two to six times higher than in the general population [3], with an early peak in the first year after cancer treatment, probably due to pre-existing heart disease, the toxicity of the treatment and the cardiotoxicity of the tumour itself [4]. Thereafter, there is a chronic phase, during which cardiovascular mortality increases over the years. The risk of cardiovascular death varies according to the different types of cancer. The added value of cardio-oncology lies in personalised management, based on the specific characteristics of the patient and the tumour.

The aim of creating a cardio oncology unit is to :

-Detect the cardiovascular complications of cancer and malignant haemopathy, and initiate treatment in good time.

- Diagnosing and managing heart failure in relation to oncology treatments.
- Diagnosing and managing vascular diseases in connection with oncology treatments.

The aim of cardio-oncology is therefore to prepare patients adequately (prevention), support them (detection) and treat them rapidly before, during and after their cancer treatment. Good collaboration between oncologists/hematologists and cardiologists remains essential in this respect. At the level of our cardiology department, faced with an ever-increasing number of cancer patients, the complexity and medical supervision they require have led us to devise services provided within a cardio-oncology unit.

In this work, we will look at the design of the project to set up a cardio-oncology unit in our department, as well as its academic prospects in terms of training students and nursing staff.

The aim is to :

1- identify the needs of the cardiology department for the creation of a cardio-oncology unit.

2-Setting up a cardio-oncology unit.

3-Draw up a plan for setting up a cardio-oncology unit, describing the various stages and resources required.

Methods

To design this project, we followed a **QQOQCCP** plan (What, Who, Where, When, How, How much and Why?) represented by **5 project sheets.**

The ishikawa diagram was used to identify the various problems.

The working group will be made up of the head of the cardiology department, the cardiologist (project director), the oncologist (project co-director), the hematologist (project co-director) and the nurse (cardio-oncology coordinator), as well as collaborating cardiologists (rhythmologist, interventional cardiologist, echocardiographist, etc.).

The SWOT (Strength, Weakness, Opportunities, Threats) method was used to study our project's chances of success.

The GANT diagram: Drawing up a roadmap.

The Deming Wheel was used to evaluate the project.

As part of the **university component** of this project, we intend to develop the skills of our trainees in patient care:

- full information about the clinical examination and additional tests that will be carried out during the consultation.
- therapeutic education about the cardiotoxic complications that can arise during or after anticancer treatment, and the need for regular monitoring to detect and treat them in good time.

Results

Cardiovascular side-effects are increasingly frequent in cancer patients undergoing cardio-toxic treatments, firstly because of the growing prevalence of this pathology, and secondly because of the development of its therapeutic arsenal and, consequently, an improvement in their survival. The result is an ever-increasing demand for cardiological consultations, echo-cardiographic examinations and appropriate therapeutic management, all of which are increasing exponentially.

As a result, the creation of a cardio oncology unit seems necessary in order to provide appropriate, well-coded therapeutic management for these fragile patients.

To analyse the difficulties involved in managing these patients, we **drew** up an **ISHIKAWA** cause-and-effect **diagram**, providing a graphic representation of a brainstorm with a summary view of the causes identified **(Figure 1)**.

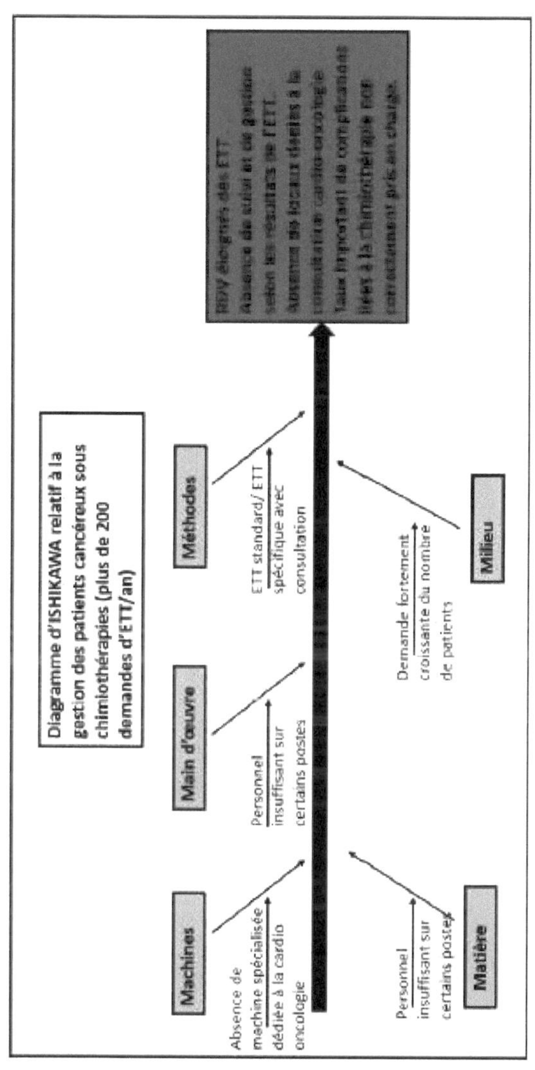

Figure 1: ISHIKAWA diagram representing the main causes identified for problems in managing cancer patients receiving cardio-toxic treatment.

CHAPTER 1

1. PROJECT SHEET 1: WHY: CURRENT SITUATION / RATIONALE / OBJECTIVES?

Before any consideration could be given to developing a cardio-oncology unit, it was imperative to first carry out an assessment of the existing situation.

Quantitative diagnosis: using indicators to assess outpatient activity

- Number of requests for cardio oncology consultations per week ;
- Number of requests for emergency cardiological assessment per week ;
- Number of requests for transthoracic echocardiography per week ;
- Number of hospital admissions for outpatient treatment per week ;
- Cancellation rate on D0 (cancellation on the scheduled day of the consultation) ;
- Maximum possible activity from the echocardiography room and offline study software (echo PAC) dedicated to cardio-oncology.

Qualitative diagnosis: assessing the organisation and maturity of the school in terms of a number of areas:

- Resources / means ;
- Management and tools ;
- Care pathway.

To do this, we evaluated outpatient activity in transthoracic echocardiography performed as part of chemotherapy (pre-, per- or post-cure) **in the absence of a dedicated unit**. This evaluation enabled us to establish the following statistics **(Figure 2)**.

We used the non-invasive exploration unit's data management software to carry out a survey along these lines. This enabled us to estimate the **proportion of requests for echocardiography/year in the context of monitoring a patient undergoing chemotherapy carried out in our department at around 9%**.

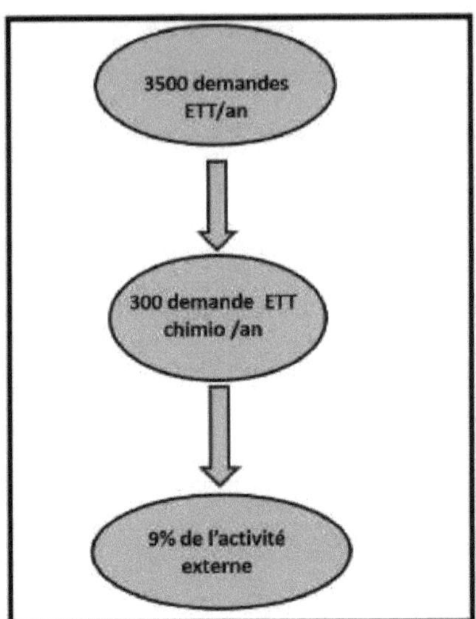

Figure 2: Cardio-oncology activity in the context of chemotherapy without a dedicated cardio-oncology unit (average annual figures between 2019 and 2020)

Furthermore, these statistics underestimate the number of requests because they do not take into account patients referred to the cardiology consultation for assessment after treatment or during cardio-toxic treatment. Furthermore, these echocardiograms performed as part of anti-cancer treatment did not take into account the patient as a whole, who did not benefit from either an overall assessment or therapeutic management tailored to each specific clinical situation.

The lack of premises dedicated to this specialised cardio oncology activity was particularly problematic with :

- **the absence of a** well-coded **patient pathway** (essential in this context, where rigorous organisation of the procedures scheduled during the day requires perfect coordination between the various players and the patient);
- **the absence of dedicated staff** with specific training in this area of care, which requires a high level of expertise to avoid the pitfalls.

Because of its volume and annual extension, this major activity has caused a significant reduction in the normal activity of the echocardiography laboratory and conventional care units, due to the overcrowding caused by patients who are often tired and frail in this context, and who do not benefit from a comprehensive cardiological assessment because they do not have a dedicated unit.

CHAPTER 2

II. PROJECT SHEET 2: WHAT, WHERE AND HOW? PRODUCT AVAILABLE

To meet these organisational needs and provide adequate, specialised care, the priority is to create a **cardio-oncology unit.**

11.1. Definition of the cardio-oncology unit

This is a structured hospital unit capable of providing specialised care for patients undergoing anti-cancer treatments, mainly: a cardiology consultation, an echocardiography and, depending on the indications, another non-invasive investigation; and, if necessary, a short stay in hospital of less than 12 hours (from 8 am to 6 pm) for patients proposed for an invasive diagnostic and/or therapeutic procedure in cardiology (e.g. coronary angiography, coronary angioplasty, programmed external electric shock, etc.).).

11.2. Purpose and scope of the structure

This is an alternative to conventional hospitalisation for medical cardiology, with a focus on short-term care:

- Essentially a cardiological consultation (questioning, clinical examination, electrocardiogram)
- But also certain non-invasive explorations: echocardiography transthoracic, Holter rhythm, Holter blood pressure and stress test.
- Short hospitalisation for patients proposed for an invasive procedure diagnostic and/or therapeutic in cardiology.

11.3. Description of the medical structure

The cardio oncology unit will have 6 inpatient beds.

During this **operational phase** of the design of our cardio-oncology unit, we are going to describe the **spatial organisation**, describing the main sectors/activity areas that have been used as **architectural recommendations**.

This organisation is based mainly on the availability and modularity of supports (bed, armchair-bed), thus optimising patient rotation. The list of rooms required for the unit to function properly is set out in **Table 1** and includes

Table 1: Structural requirements at the architectural level in terms of

premises to be considered.

Cardio-Oncology Unit	
Home	
Home	1
Waiting	1
Sanitary	2
Multi-purpose office	1
Consultation office	1
Echocardiography room	1
Inpatient unit	
Patient changing rooms - Undressing cubicles	2
Lounge - meals	1
Individual boxes	7
Patient toilet blocks	3
Nursing station	1
- Administrative area (shared area)	
- Preparation / care (shared area)	1
Medical-technical logistics	
Storage of rolling stock (stretchers)	1
Small equipment storage	1
Food office	1
Clean linen	1
Dirty laundry - waste	1
Housekeeping	1
Relaxation room - staff	1
Staff toilets	2

11.3.1. Reception area

The reception will be structured around the following areas:

- **Reception - executive / secretariat:** enables administrative formalities to be completed where necessary.
- **Medical/carer interview office:** on arrival, the patient is either sent directly from

reception to the care area, or received for a cardio-oncological consultation. This is started by a nurse, who takes vital parameters and performs an electrocardiogram. The doctor then performs a cardiology consultation with a transthoracic echocardiography and validates outpatient treatment if required.

11.3.2. Patient care premises

Table 2: Architectural composition of this hospital unit.

Architecture required	Number
Reception room	1
Doctors' offices	3
Cloakroom	1
Hospitalisation room	1
Inpatient beds with scope	6
Catheter room	1
Ultrasound room	1
Resuscitation trolley	1

- Patient monitoring: a nurse's office for preparation and care will be consider.

II.3.3. Medical and technical logistics" premises :

- **Storage:** for large and small items (stretchers, wheelchairs);
- **Logistics:** for clean linen, dirty linen, waste and cleaning;
- **Staff relaxation, changing rooms:** to be adapted according to the organisation of the service.

11.4. Continuation of care :

During its opening hours (8am to 6pm), the cardio oncology unit is committed to ensuring the continuity of patient care through the permanent presence of medical, paramedical and social staff.

An extreme emergency procedure will be posted in the treatment room and known to all.

The mobile numbers of the various doctors will also be displayed.

In addition, the cardio-oncology unit will be located close to the cardiac intensive care unit.

Outside opening hours, the cardiology department has beds for conventional hospitalisation and intensive care, where patients can be referred if necessary (procedural complications, acute heart failure following anti-cancer treatment, etc.).

11.5. Organisation and patient flow

11.5.1. Mission of the cardio-oncology unit

The cardio-oncology unit: the same indications and organisational requirements in terms of diagnosis and therapy. The procedures are carried out in units that are part of the cardiology department or the hospital: medical imaging, interventional catheterisation (functional explorations), non-invasive cardiological explorations, various medical opinions (oncology, pharmacology, endocrinology, neurology, pneumology, gastroenterology, cardiac surgery, etc.). The main differences between this mode of operation and a conventional hospital service are :

- The recruitment of patients who are **pre-included in a care circuit** with **a programme of pre-established examinations or procedures.**
- By identifying patients who may require hospitalisation, depending on the type of procedure proposed and the medical and social criteria relating to the patient,
- And lastly, the need for comprehensive patient care to enable

same-day patient discharge.

However, despite the attention paid to prior assessment of these patients, continued hospitalisation in a conventional hospital or ICU is sometimes necessary.

11.5.2. Patient origin :

- Consultant oncologists in the hospital, either referring patients who have been followed for a long time, or patients who have chosen our hospital for a diagnostic procedure.
- Hematologists, surgeons, internists or any doctor referring patients who will require anti-cancer treatment.

11.5.3. Patient care according to the reason for consultation

Outpatient care in the cardio-oncology unit will be organised according to the following essential stages:

11.5.3.1. Consultation :

- A consultation appointment (RDV) will have to be made by the patient using a detailed pre-established form (see appendix 1), usually completed by an oncologist.
- The patient will undergo a full cardiovascular examination (interview, clinical examination, electrocardiogram) (appendix 2) with a specialised transthoracic echocardiogram (appendix 3).

11.5.3.2. The patient is admitted to the cardio-oncology unit with rapid initial management:

- At medical level, analysis of the case history, clinical examination and ECG to guide therapeutic management.
- At paramedical level, additional biological tests if necessary, placement of an approach, information, scope if necessary.

Patient discharge

- The social criteria will be checked: relatives at home, time off work, return home accompanied, call for a registered taxi or ambulance.
- The hospitalisation report is drawn up for inclusion in the department's database and, where appropriate, for sending to the oncologist and the attending physician as a minimum.
- Patients and their families will be given as much information as possible.
- The patient will be given a discharge summary and the reports of additional examinations.
- Presentation of the file to the monthly multidisciplinary staff of the cardio-oncology unit, including : cardiologist, oncologist, hematologist,

pharmacist and psychologist, and a consultation with the patient will be organised if necessary.

- A telephone call to the treating oncologist or doctor will be considered if consultation is necessary.

11.5.3.3. In the event of transfer to conventional hospitalisation

- Agreement with the doctors in charge of the patient thereafter.
- Prescription biology and treatment.
- The discharge and the prescription will be signed by the doctors in charge of the patient the following day; the discharge prescription, which has been prepared but not given to the patient, can therefore be amended if necessary.

II.6. Medicinal treatment

They will be asked to come to the cardio oncology unit with their prescriptions and various treatments.

The treatment will be reviewed and prescribed by the doctor on the basis of the results of the clinical examinations. The treatment is then prepared by the nurse and the medication is kept in the treatment room to be returned to the patient on discharge.

II.7. Medical file

11.6.1. Drawing up a medical file

The patient's medical file in the cardio-oncology unit is a paper file which will be archived in a dedicated space in the cardio-oncology archive.

Each doctor called upon to provide care, give an opinion, propose treatment or take a therapeutic decision is solely responsible for drafting the information relating to his or her actions.

Keeping medical records is the responsibility of every doctor who takes charge of a patient.

11.6.2. Archiving medical records

The nursing staff compile the patient's file and send it to the secretariat for archiving.

In fact, the file will only be definitively archived once certain tests have been carried out and any decisions taken by the multidisciplinary staff have been taken into account.

All measures will be taken to ensure the safekeeping and confidentiality of the files kept in the department.

11.6.3. **Communication of medical records**

Reports of additional examinations will be given to the patient.

A hospital report is sent as soon as possible to the oncologist or doctor in charge of the patient (<7 days) unless a decision or examination is pending.

The oncologist or any other doctor involved will be contacted whenever necessary.

A multidisciplinary team will be set up periodically to make the right decisions in difficult cases.

CHAPTER 3

III. PROJECT SHEET 3: WHO? HUMAN RESOURCES

No recruitment is planned at strategic human resources level. Redeployment of medical and paramedical staff will be envisaged according to the requirements of the following job profiles **(figure 3)**:

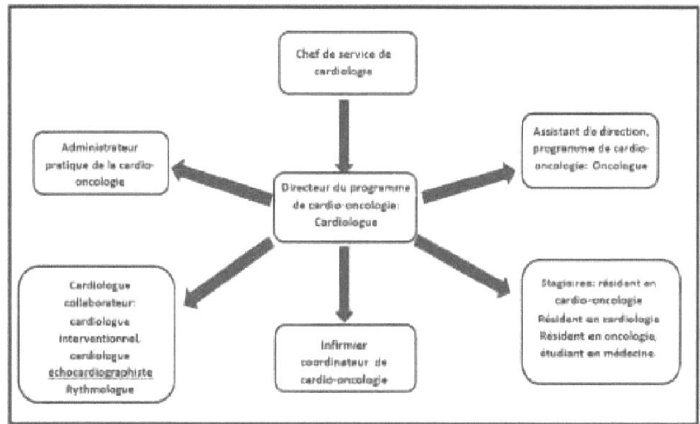

<u>Figure 3: Organisation of the medical and paramedical team at Cardio-oncological activity</u>

111.1. <u>Coordinating cardiologist :</u>

Supervision of the organisation of the service by a coordinating doctor who is genuinely committed and available, responsible for steering the structure and working with the teams to improve the synchronisation of the different players' work with patients:

- Unit coordination,

Validation of requests for day hospitalisation for certain patients for whom the relevance of day hospitalisation is debatable (heart failure, suspected coronary artery disease, rhythm disorder, significant valvulopathy, etc.),

- Monitoring activity indicators and quality of care,
- Setting up a network of corresponding GPs

(telephone, post, e-mail),

- Update and discussion of the management of each patient

multidisciplinary staff if necessary.

111.2. Coordinating oncologist :

Executive assistant to the cardio-oncologist in this unit; he is also the one who indicates and chooses the anti-cancer treatment for each patient according to the recommendations of the learned societies.

111.3. Resident (1 full-time equivalent)

Medical monitoring of the patient, with the patient's care adapted in consultation with the coordinating doctor.

Residents assigned to the cardio oncology unit will be expected to take part in the unit's medical activities.

111.4. Nurse :

What's special about this unit from a nursing point of view is that the nursing team takes complete charge of the patient, organising the day's schedule in the cardio-oncology unit, informing the patient, welcoming him or her, monitoring the day's progress and discharging him or her. In addition, the nurses working in 12-hour shifts ensure that each patient receives continuous care, which adds consistency and avoids loss of time and information between teams.

The tasks of the nursing team will be :

- Preparation for hospitalisation, telephone reception of correspondents and telephone and postal notification of patients, with delivery of the necessary instructions,
- On arrival, welcoming and settling in patients, checking and completing check-ups if necessary, inserting a venous line, shaving and hygiene care, issuing medication prescribed by the facility, contact with the anaesthetist, catheter room and examination rooms,
- Patient care on return,
- Monitoring (including, but not limited to, vital signs, pain according to the visual analogue scale, puncture site, electrocardiogram, re-dressing of arterial and/or venous compression dressings)
- Organising discharge, making appointments and providing discharge documents,

transferring patients to conventional hospital care (in collaboration with the department's managers) with transmission of the nursing file; providing information to patients (therapeutic education++) and their families.

- Delivery of treatments in accordance with the medical prescription, updated according to the procedure performed,
- Meal management also depends on the examinations carried out,
- Social assessment to help organise the return home
- In addition, the nurses are responsible for maintaining a medicine cabinet containing the products needed to prepare patients prior to procedures carried out in the day hospital, and for monitoring and updating resuscitation equipment, including a resuscitation trolley and a defibrillator.

111.5. <u>Supervisor:</u>

Whose activity will be shared between the different sectors (consultation sector, non-invasive or invasive functional explorations and the inpatient part of the unit).

111.6. <u>Medical secretary :</u>

<u>An efficient secretariat</u> will manage the flow of information and schedule appointments. It will constantly seek the best use of the various resources, draw up summaries of documents (required for the care pathway), and pass on information to the various parties involved (including patients) inside and outside the hospital. This is the same secretary in charge of the functional investigations unit. Her specific duties will include:

- Entering and sending mail to the attending physician using the department's computerised reporting software
- Entering activity indicators
- Keeping patient records

- Recovery of medical documents obtained after the patient has been discharged and requiring specific archiving (reports of interventional, imaging and biological procedures, etc.)

111.7. <u>Social worker (occasionally)</u>

111.8. <u>Dietician (on call, not assigned to the facility)</u>

111.9. <u>Psychologist (on call, not assigned to the facility)</u>

Discussion

Our discussion will address 3 constraints to the project, relating to :

- The context in which it was created, with the conditions, interferences and possible dependencies,
- The resources that will be allocated to it,
- We are also looking into the possibility of developing this unit into a university unit, where cancer patients receive optimal care.

1. **PROJECT SHEET 4: WHERE? IN WHAT CONTEXT? STUDY OF THE RELEVANCE AND COHERENCE OF THE PROJECT**

1.1. **Terms and conditions**

The cardio oncology unit should enable patients to stay in hospital for a few hours to receive the care they need before returning to their place of residence. The essential prerequisites for this project are :

1.1.1. **Heritage and architecture**

We quickly found ourselves faced with a number of architectural constraints, with decisions to be made regarding the **conversion of a non-invasive functional exploration unit into an outpatient cardio-oncology unit** or the **construction of new areas**. This conversion will be carried out after validation by the experts and architects.

- **Patients and carers:**

It is important to note that invasive cardiology procedures (cardiac catheterisation, rhythmology procedures, etc.) carried out on an outpatient basis reduce mobility, leading to a loss of autonomy and difficulty in driving, carrying heavy loads, grooming, etc., particularly in the case of fragile patients undergoing anti-cancer treatments...

There are often a large number of people (usually the patient's relatives) accompanying the patient during treatment and on discharge, and they need to be taken into account in the waiting areas, in order to facilitate the flow of admissions and discharges.

- **Staff :**

Staff in several categories (doctors, nurses, care assistants, medical secretaries, etc.)

working as a team will be put to good use in the cardio-oncology unit.

So, when restructuring, the quest for economic efficiency will have to be combined with two issues that must also remain at the heart of project managers' ambitions, namely :

- Optimising conditions for patients and their carers;
- Respect for privacy and confidentiality in the open-plan unit (lounge) and the separate design of a "women's" room.
- Ergonomics, functionality and quality of life at work for all the professionals working in this structure.

1.1.2. Dedicated and experienced team

The formation of a **dedicated** team**, experienced in** the management of patients, which has previously drawn up clinical pathways for the unit's homogeneous group of prevalent patients, with the aim of **planning, organising and ensuring** the consensual management of patients. A number of parameters need to be taken into account before, during and after hospitalisation, so that patients can be discharged on the same day as a trained team, in compliance with strict safety criteria, particularly after coronary angioplasty.

1.1.3. Preparing a pre-established but personalised patient pathway

The patient pathway comprises the following stages:

1. Consultation with echocardiography specialised
2. Pre-admission (if any)
3. The previous day's call
4. Welcoming and caring for patients in the unit
5. The catheter room and post-intervention monitoring

(coronary angiography, angioplasty, interventional rhythmology, etc.)

6. Post-operative patient care and monitoring
7. Therapeutic patient education.
8. The patient's actual discharge

A specialised consultation, including a transthoracic echocardiogram, is the key step in ensuring that the patient's treatment progresses smoothly. Consultation with the paramedical teams (nurses, social workers, psychologist) may be necessary. The **patient** must **confirm that he/she** agrees with the treatment plan.

The patient's state of health and autonomy must be assessed beforehand. If hospitalisation is indicated, it should only be carried out as part of a healthcare network involving the attending cardiologist, the attending physician, the local medical analysis laboratory and the patient's family and friends.

1.1.4. Simple, easy-to-read accessibility within the establishment

The general organisation of the various circuits or flows (patients, professionals, equipment and information) must be reviewed and made accessible. The cardio-oncology unit must be easily accessible, with appropriate signage.

1.1.5. Continuous care

Following a planned hospitalisation in a cardio-oncology unit, discharge is planned for the same day, but will require follow-up by telephone the following day for the sub-category of patients who have benefited from outpatient angioplasty, to check for any complications. All patients will have their renal function checked at 48 hours by telephone, fax or e-mail.

I.2. Interfering factors and dependencies

The strategic study and the decision to set up this project were based on an analysis of its relevance and coherence. A summary phase was therefore carried out, with the formalisation of a **SWOT-type matrix** describing the project's strengths, weaknesses, opportunities and threats. This analysis will enable the project to maximise its assets (strengths and opportunities) and minimise its weaknesses (weaknesses and threats).

The evaluation was carried out in 2 stages to identify the internal factors that could be modified and the external factors that could interfere with the success of the project and its sustainable development **(Figure 4)**.

SWOT ANALYSIS

Forces

- Équipe médicale et paramédicale expérimentée et formée
- Absence de nouvelles constructions (reconversion des locaux) ni de recrutement (redéploiement de l'effectif)
- Parcours patient défini et spécialisé.

Faiblesses

L'absence de prise de rendez-vous précis dans le temps (inadéquation des horaires de démarrage et d'arrivé du malade).
Engorgement des patients attendant les explorations au niveau de la salle d'attente.
Longue attente pour la paperasse administrative.

Opportunités

- Augmentation de la demande de suivi cardiologique des patients cancéreux sous traitement.
- Projet de réaménagement du service.
- Motivation des oncologues et des hématologues de l'hôpital pour ce projet.
- Prise en charge optimisé du patient cancéreux sous traitement cardio-toxique.

Menaces

- L'absence de prise de rendez-vous précis dans le temps (inadéquation des horaires de démarrage et d'arrivé du malade).
- Engorgement des patients attendant les explorations au niveau de la salle d'attente.
- Longue attente pour la paperasse administrative.
- Complexité de la décision thérapeutique (arrêt de la chimiothérapie++)

Forces

* experienced and well-trained medical and paramedical team
* No new buildings (conversion of premises) or recruitment (redeployment of workforce)
* Definite and specialist patient pathway.

Opportunities

* Increasing demand for cardiological follow-up of cancer patients undergoing treatment.
* Department reorganisation project.
* Motivation for the project from the hospital's oncologists and haematologists.
* Optimal management of cancer patients undergoing cardiotoxic treatment.

Weaknesses

Failure to make precise appointments (inadequate start and arrival times).

Overcrowding of patients waiting for explorations in the waiting room.

Long wait for administrative paperwork.

Lack of precise appointment times (mismatch between the patient's arrival and departure times).

Overcrowding of patients waiting for explorations in the waiting room.

Long wait for administrative paperwork.

Complexity of the therapeutic decision (stopping chemotherapy++)

Figure 4: SWOT matrix (Strengths, Weaknesses, Opportunities, Threats) for the strategic analysis of the project to set up a cardio-oncology unit.

- Among the technological innovations that have improved the management of cancer patients is a new imaging technique called longitudinal strain, which is myocardial deformation where (Strain)= is the expression of the change in length of a segment and can be written as follows: E=L-L°/L° where L° is the initial length of the myocardial fibre and L its length after deformation. It is **expressed as a percentage.** It represents a promising tool for the early detection of ventricular dysfunction and has shown its value in several studies[6-9] **(Figure 5+6):**

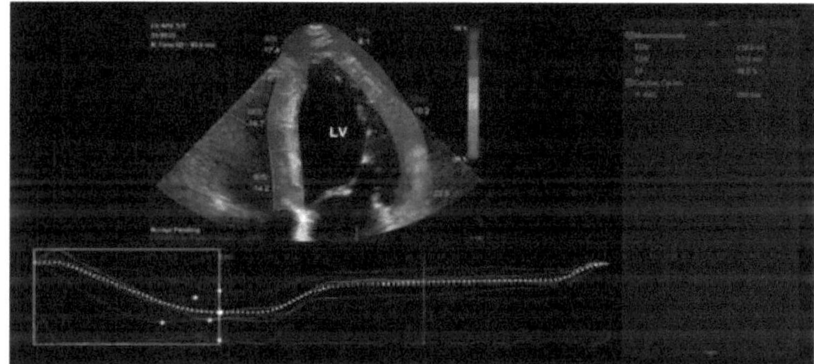

Figure 5: Myocardial deformation imaging showing the stained LV wall with segmental subdivision, allowing reassessment of segmental strain but, more importantly, reassessment of LV volumes and ejection fraction.

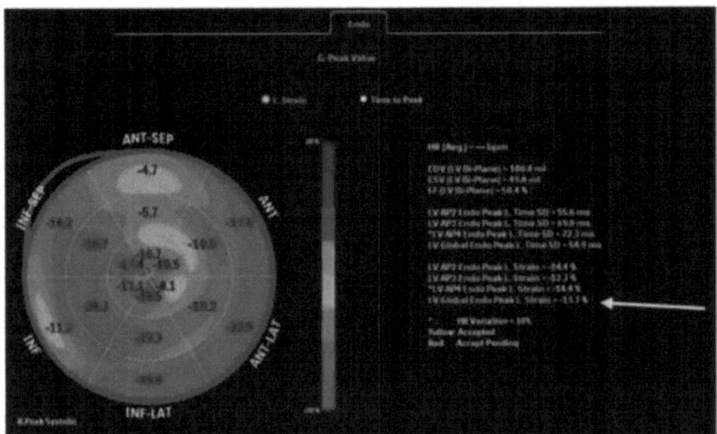

<u>Figure 6: Bull's eye of the global longitudinal strain with the strain value of each segment associated with a colour code according to the value.</u>

II. PROJECT SHEET 5: HOW MUCH? WHEN?

We are going to try to control the investment in terms of time and money for this project.

The spatial conversion of the non-invasive functional exploration unit will be adopted for this project.

A design office will establish the architectural, technical and financial requirements of the project.

The multidisciplinary cardio-oncology team with expertise in the management of cancer patients with co-morbidities, such as heart disease, appears to be more effective than doctors working without a dedicated cardio-oncology unit. Cancer patients with asthma, diabetes, chronic renal failure or heart failure benefited from a more global and comprehensive approach to care. A meta-analysis of randomised trials involving patients with heart failure showed that cardio-oncology units are associated with a reduction in mortality and hospitalisations [9]. Multidisciplinary teams should improve coordination, communication and decision-making between members of the healthcare team and patients, and help to improve the management of these patients [10].

To optimise the installation schedule for this new unit and limit the time required for the work, a **GANTT diagram** (see appendices) will be drawn up to help manage the various parties involved.

III. PROJECT ASSESSMENT

This evaluation component will aim to improve the quality of care for cancer patients. Both quantitative and qualitative indicators (relating to patient satisfaction) will be adopted.

It will take place in 4 phases, represented schematically by the **DEMING WHEEL (Figure 7).**

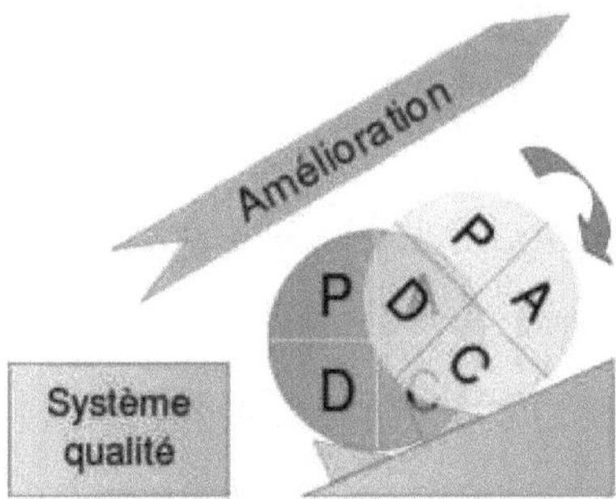

Figure 7: Deming wheel representing the 4 stages: Plan, Do, Check and Act, of the quality system that will be put in place for the project to set up a cardio-oncology unit.

The method comprises four stages, each leading to the next, and aims to establish a virtuous circle by capitalising on the knowledge acquired.

- **Plan:** Plan and prepare the work to be done. Setting objectives

Define the tasks to be carried out. Specify the tasks and responsibilities. Above all, don't forget to specify the performance criteria. As part of the analysis of the populations cared for within the establishment, specific care for cancer patients was defined. The risk analysis of the patient pathway process was coordinated at institutional level by the steering group, and at operational level by the director and co-director of the cardio-oncology unit.

- **Do: To** do, to carry out, to perform the tasks planned. It can be

It's a good idea to limit the size and scope of the tasks to be carried out in order to have better control (repetitive process). A short project is easier to manage and, without fear of overstatement, delivers results more quickly. You can then better redirect the rest of the project, whatever it may be. Internal organisation ensures that resources, and in particular skills, are matched to the needs of the care provided. The specialist skills required for patient care are identified. The lists and contact details of all specialist doctors are drawn up and made available to all the professionals concerned. The health care organisation has identified the situations and patients requiring education in the form of either a personalised programme or targeted educational activities enabling patients to participate in the follow-up to treatment and care at the end of their stay. The premises are adapted to the activities carried out and the needs of the patients. The premises, equipment and materials benefit from an effective preventive and curative maintenance system. The system for dealing with life-threatening emergencies is adapted and organised: the list of on-call specialists and their contact details are drawn up, displayed and known to professionals. Monthly multi-disciplinary meetings enable the care plan to be constantly readjusted and care plans to be monitored. These are drawn up and personalised for each patient, incorporating a benefit-risk approach. Patients are discharged in such a way as to ensure continuity and safety of care: a letter from the attending physician, prescriptions needed to continue treatment and monitoring, and follow-up appointments.

✓ **Check:** to verify the results. Measuring and comparing with forecasts. This is the key to continuous improvement. The check phase isn't just a time for handing out medals and kicks. It's when you realise how difficult (or simple) a given task is. It's also the time when you learn to control your forecasts more effectively, so it's essential to take regular stock of patient turnover and identify areas for improvement;

✓ To analyse the various stages in the patient's journey, starting with the cardio-oncology consultation; making the appointment, waiting time and, secondly, as an outpatient in the health establishment and on the day of the operation: arrival, reception, registration, preparation, operation in the catheter room or rhythm room, discharge, rehabilitation, assessment of "streetability", care by the accompanying person;

✓ Identify any blockages in the circuit that prevent a fixed target rotation rate;

Act: Act, correct, take the necessary decisions. Identify the causes of deviations between what was achieved and what was expected. Identify new points of intervention, redefine processes if necessary. Improvement actions are carried out following the results of the various evaluation and risk analysis actions. The Quality and Risk Management coordinator works with the pilot working group to update the action plans. The results are communicated at departmental meetings by the managers appointed for each action in the action plan.

IV. ACADEMIC ASPECT OF THE PROJECT

The **academic component of** this cardio-oncology unit, which will be offered to medical externs, but also to the nursing team to be trained, interns and residents, with different objectives in terms of the taxonomic levels to be achieved, will include, among other things, examples of the following activities linked to the area of **knowledge and skills.**

The patient circuit in this unit includes:

- an initial contact or an important stage in the treatment consists of providing **information and obtaining informed consent**;
- a second contact after a cardiovascular assessment and specialised trans-thoracic echocardiography, where **therapeutic education** is essential to ensure compliance with treatment and control of cardiovascular risk factors.

To achieve this, two sessions of one to one-and-a-half hours of **role-play teaching** will be provided for each group of students. This teaching will be assessed by **structured objective clinical evaluation stations**.

IV.1 Definition of a role-playing game

Role-playing is a teaching technique for learning interpersonal skills.

The aim is to simulate a situation which is likely to occur but which is not always predictable. People play a more or less determined role, improvising the dialogue [1113].

IV.2 Advantages of role-playing

In addition to theoretical knowledge (Knowledge), learning **through role-playing** will focus on interpersonal skills (enabling an aspect of professional interpersonal skills to be explored). The aim is to get to know oneself better and to adjust as a practitioner [21-23]. This group learning allows,

- To encourage sensory representations (the aim is no longer to discuss concepts or reported experiences, but to discuss experiences).
- To have a revealing effect on problems linked to verbal and non-verbal communication.
- Encourage learning by linking the familiar with the new.

- Reinforcing the integration of knowledge by making participants players.
- It can be combined with video, and one of its main advantages is "autoscopy": it allows you to discover your own behaviour and actively train new behaviours.

IV.3 Conduct of the session

This teaching technique requires strict rules to be observed, both when planning the game and during the three stages: before, during and after the game.

The role of the patient can be played by another participant, by the facilitator or the expert, or by an outsider trained to play this role according to a specific scenario (standardised patient).

For each session, there will be 2 teachers, one of whom will be the facilitator and the other will be the "expert" who can be consulted if a problem arises during the game. This two-teacher organisation will enable the full benefits of the technique to be enjoyed and the pitfalls to be avoided [21-23].

Scenario and procedure for role-playing sessions

The artificial situation will be written down in advance by the teachers. During each of the role-play sessions, the students will be informed of the type of teaching that will take place, without knowing the precise situation that will be addressed.

The session will last between **1h and 1h30**. The procedure will be as follows [21-23] :

- **Preparation: 10 to 20 minutes:** this will be used to set up a scene based on concrete situations around the 2 set themes. A reminder of the rules of the game will be given. This phase is essential for the rest of the performance. A distribution of roles will be proposed by the protagonists. The camera will be taken over by a member of the group who is not taking part in the game.
- **The role-play itself: 20 minutes:**
- **Discussion (debriefing): 30 to 40 minutes:** between students and teacher facilitators.
- Start with the experience of the actors,

- The audience is then given the floor, within the limits of the subject, to make their own observations and interpretations.

- **The role of the facilitator:** The facilitator facilitates and regulates the work of the group when the scenario is being set up. After the game, he/she supports the analysis of the different elements of the game.

The role-play sessions will be described in advance through interviews conducted by experts with real patients or through video-recorded illustration. Examples of different situations with the different items to be addressed are shown in the following grids.

Example 1: You are treating Mr HA, aged 60, who is a smoker and diabetic on ADO for left ventricular dysfunction following cardio-toxic chemotherapy treatment. He is due to undergo coronary angiography. He contacts you because he has had no information about this examination, which he is apprehensive about. He is asking you about the benefits of the test and how it will be carried out.

Why is this?

1. Explain the clinical presentation and the coronary involvement (narrowing or or occlusion).
2. Establish a precise lesion assessment and propose the appropriate treatment.
3. Can lead to :

- medical treatment
- angioplasty
- coronary artery bypass grafting

4. Improving symptoms and/or survival

How does it work?

1. Performed under local anaesthetic, painless.
2. X-ray examination
3. Cardiac catheterization by arterial puncture arterial puncture

4. Opacification of the coronary arteries <u>with iodine contrast medium</u>

Greeting at the beginning and end, introducing yourself Reassuring the patient

Example 2: You are treating Mrs FK for cardiotoxic treatment. You advise her to take up physical activity. She asks you about the possible benefits of this activity.

When will it take place?

During or after the course of chemotherapy **Interets?**

Improvement of :

1. Cardiorespiratory function.
2. Body composition (preservation

or increase in muscle mass, reduction in fat mass).

3. The immune function.
4. Muscular strength
5. Body image, self-esteem

Reduction of :

1. The frequency and severity of the undesirable effects of chemotherapy, such as nausea, fatigue and pain.
2. The length of hospitalisation.
3. Stress, depression and anxiety. **Greeting at the beginning and end, introducing yourself Reassuring the patient**

Conclusions

Cancer is a public health problem in Tunisia. Projections for 2024, based on the cancer register for northern Tunisia, indicate that the standardised incidence of all cancer sites in men will rise from 143.3 per 100,000 individuals for the period 2004-2008 to 184.2 for the period 2019-2024 [20]. The improvement in cancer survival has led to a growing number of Tunisians being affected by cancer on the one hand, and by cardiovascular disease on the other. It is therefore vital to organise specific cardiovascular monitoring for patients who are due to receive treatment that is potentially toxic to the cardiovascular system. This is the background to the emergence of cardio-oncology, whose main objective is to prevent, detect and manage cardiovascular disease associated with or secondary to anti-cancer treatment without compromising its efficacy. Analysis of the current situation at the main military training hospital in Tunis has revealed a number of shortcomings in the management of consultation appointments, explorations and therapeutic management of cancer patients, who are increasingly frequent and fragile.

At the same time, multidisciplinary cardio-oncology programmes need to be developed to improve patient care.

For these reasons, we are proposing the creation of a cardio-oncology unit in cardiology at the military hospital, where patients will be able to benefit from clear, standardised care programmes, especially as they are increasingly numerous and complex, with multi-system involvement, and provide access to high-quality consultations and complementary cardiovascular examinations as quickly as possible, so as not to delay cancer treatment by minimising cardiovascular risks. What's more, if necessary, patients can benefit from a short stay in hospital, during which we will perform a coronary angiography and/or angioplasty, followed by a few hours of monitoring.

Conclusions

This document provides the key elements for the major change in practice represented by the cardio-oncology unit, a change made possible by the multidisciplinary team, which is improving coordination, communication and decision-making in cancer patients in order to prevent, detect and manage the cardiovascular toxicity of anti-cancer treatments in good time.

At the same time, we explored the possibilities of maintaining an academic vocation in this unit. For example, role-playing scenarios were devised to teach patients how to inform themselves on admission about any invasive examinations that might be indicated, and to provide them with therapeutic education on discharge.

References

[1] Benjamin E.J, Muntner P, Alonso A,et al. Heart disease and stroke statistics-2019 update.Circulation.2019; 139, e56-e528.

[2] Zamorano JL, Lancellotti P, Munoz DR, AboyansV, Asteggiano R, Galderisi M et al. ESC Position Paper on cancer treatments and cardiovascular toxicity developed under the auspices of the ESC Committee for Practice Guidelines The Task Force for cancer treatments and cardiovascular toxicity of the European Society of Cardiology (ESC). Eur Heart J.2016; 37 (36), 2768-2801

[3] Sturgeon KM, Deng L, Bluethmann SM, Zhou S, Trifiletti DM, Jiang C et al. A population-based study of cardiovascular disease mortality risk in US cancer patients. Eur Heart J. 2019 ;1-9O

[4] Herrmann, J. From trends to transformation: where cardio-oncology is to make a difference. Eur Heart J, 2019, 40 (48), 3898-3900

[5] Celutkiene J, Pudil R, Lopez-Fernandez T, Grapsa J, Nihoyannopoulos P, Bergler-Klein J et al. Role of cardiovascular imaging in cancer patients receiving cardiotoxic therapies: a position statement on behalf of the Heart Failure Association (HFA), the European Association of Cardiovascular Imaging (EACVI) and the Cardio-Oncology Council of the European Society of Cardiology (ESC). Eur J Heart Fail. 2020;22(9):1504-1524.

[6] Moslehi JJ, Witteles RM. Global Longitudinal Strain in Cardio-Oncology. J Am Coll Cardiol. 2021;77(4):402-404

[7] Thavendiranathan P, Poulin F, Lim KD, Plana JC, Woo A, Marwick TH. Use of myocardial strain imaging by echocardiography for the early detection of cardiotoxicity in patients during and after cancer chemotherapy: a systematic review. J Am Coll Cardiol. 2014;63(25 Pt A):2751-68.

[8] Khouri MG, Ky B, Dunn G, Plappert T, Englefield V, Rabineau D, Yow E, et al. Echocardiography Core Laboratory Reproducibility of Cardiac Safety Assessments in Cardio-Oncology. J Am Soc Echocardiogr. 2018;31(3):361- 371.e3.

[9] McAlister F, Stewart S, Ferrua S, McMurray J. Multidisciplinary strategies for the management of heart failure patients at high risk for admission: A systematic review of randomized trials. J Am Coll Cardiol. 2004;44(4)810-819.

[10]Fleissig A, Jenkins V, Catt S, Fallowfield L. Multidisciplinary teams in cancer care: are they effective in the UK? Lancet Oncol. 2006;7:935-943.

[11]Girard G, Clavet D, Boule R. Planifier et animer un jeu de role profitable pour I'apprentissage. Pedagogie Medicale 2005;6:178-85. doi:10.1051/pmed:2005022.

[12]Cuenot S, Cochand P, Lanares J, Feihl F, Bonvin R, Guex P, et al. L'apport du patient simule dans I'apprentissage de la relation medecin-malade: résultats d'une évaluation preliminaire. Pedagogie Medicale 2005;6:216-24. doi:10.1051/pmed:2005026.

[13]Deffieux X, Faivre E, Frydman R, Senat M-V. Enseigner la relation medecin- malade en gynecologie obstetrique par des seances de jeu de role. /data/revues/03682315/00370003/07004279/ 2008.

[14]Heger Lazaar-Ben Gobrane, Said Hajjem, Hajer Aounallah-Skhiri, Noureddine Achour, Mohamed Hsairi. Mortality from cancer in Tunisia: calculation of years of life lost. Sante Publique. 2011 ;23:31-40

Appendices

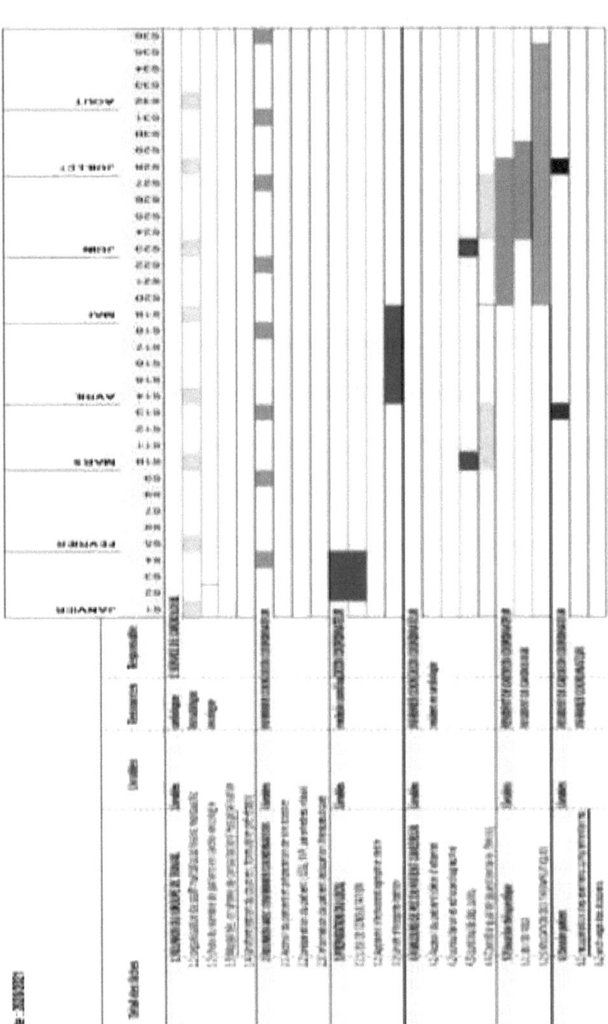

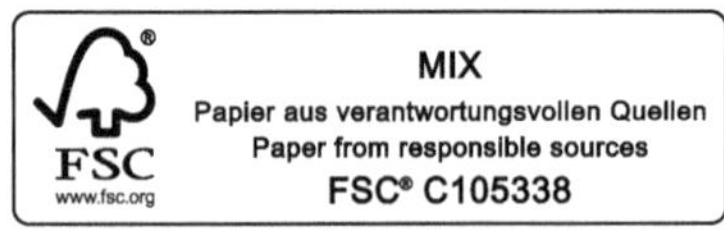

Printed by Books on Demand GmbH, Norderstedt / Germany